The Vibrant Alkaline Diet Cookbook

Amazing Alkaline Recipes to Boost Your Lifestyle and Balance Your Ph

Kris Green

Table of contents

Immunity-Boosting Soup
Preparation Time: 10 minutes

Cooking Time: 15 Minutes

Serving: 5

Ingredients

1 pack of approved-flour noodles

1 key lime

Accepted herbs

1/2 onion

1 bell pepper

Sea salt and cayenne pepper

1 cup cherry tomatoes

1 zucchini

1 cup mushrooms

1 tablespoon grapeseed oil

4 cups of water

Directions

1. Cook the noodles following the instructions.

2. Cut the onion in small dices.

3. Heat the grapeseed oil in a big pan and then sauté the onion until it's shining.

4. Cut the bell pepper, cherry tomatoes, and mushroom in small pieces.

5. Sauté this on the pan as well.

6. Also, grill the zucchini and add it to the pan.

7. Add the sea salt, pepper, spices, and water. Allow it to boil over medium heat.

8. Once it is boiled, lower the heat.

9. Then add the noodles and allow it to simmer for another 8 minutes.

10. Serve topped with key lime juice and more herbs.

Calories: 221Fat: 3.7gCarbs: 54gProtein: 6.5g Fiber: 3.5g

Blueberry-Pie Smoothie

Preparation Time: 10 minutes

Cooking Time: 15 Minutes

Serving: 3

Ingredients

1 tablespoon homemade walnut butter

1 burro banana

1/4 cup cooked amaranth

2 cups homemade soft-jelly coconut milk

1 cup fresh blueberries

1 teaspoon Bromide plus Powder

2 tablespoons date sugar

Directions

1. Blend all ingredients in your blender.

2. Let the smoothie cool in the freezer.

3. Enjoy!

Calories: 211Fat: 3.7gCarbs: 44gProtein: 6.5g Fiber: 3.5g

Alkaline-Electric Spring Salad

Preparation Time: 11 minutes

Cooking Time: 15 Minutes

Serving: 2

Ingredients

1 cup cherry tomatoes

4 cups seasonal greens

1/4 cup walnuts

1/4 cup approved herbs

For the dressing:

Sea salt and cayenne pepper

3 key limes

1 tablespoon of homemade raw sesame tahini butter

Directions

1. Sap the key limes.

2. Whisk together the homemade raw sesame "tahini" butter with the key lime juice in a small bowl.

3. Add cayenne pepper and sea salt to your satisfaction.

4. Cut the cherry tomatoes in half.

5. In a large bowl, combine the greens, cherry tomatoes, and herbs. Pour the dressing on top and massage with your hands.

6. Let the greens soak the dressing. Add more cayenne pepper, herbs, and sea salt.

7. Enjoy

Calories: 271Fat: 3.1gCarbs: 54gProtein: 6.5g Fiber: 3.5g

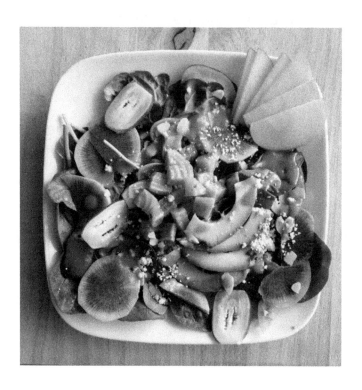

The Cleanse Juice

Preparation Time: 10 minutes

Cooking Time: 12 Minutes

Serving: 1

Ingredients

3 key limes

1/2 tsp. Bromide plus Powder

1 bunch basil or sweet basil leaves

2 cups of soft-jelly coconut water

4 seeded cucumbers

Directions

1. Juice the basil, key limes, and cucumbers.

2. Add the soft-jelly coconut water.

3. Serve the juice in a glass with the Bromide plus Powder and soft-jelly coconut water.

4. Mix well, and enjoy it!

Calories: 271Fat: 3.7gCarbs: 54gProtein: 5.5g Fiber: 3.5g

Super Hydration Smoothie

Preparation Time: 13 minutes

Cooking Time: 15 Minutes

Serving: 2

Ingredients

1 key lime, juiced

1 cup watermelon

1/2 cup soft-jelly coconut water

1/2 cup raspberries

1/4 seeded cucumber

Instructions

1. First, peel and core the cucumber and cut into tiny masses.

2. Blend all ingredients in a blender.

3. Refrigerate for 30 minutes.

4. Enjoy!

Calories: 371Fat: 3.7gCarbs: 54gProtein: 6.5g Fiber: 3.5g

Immunity-Boosting Smoothie

Preparation Time: 15 minutes

Cooking Time: 15 Minutes

Serving: 2

Ingredients

1 tablespoon date sugar or agave syrup

1 key juiced lime

1 cup brewed Alkaline Diet's Immune Support Herbal Tea

1/2 mango

1 Seville orange

1 tablespoon coconut oil

Directions

1. Heat two cups purified water and add 1½ tablespoon of Alkaline Diet's Immune Support Herbal Tea.

2. Simmer for about 15 minutes. Allow to cool, strain.

3. Peel the Seville orange and cut the mango into chunks.

4. Blend all the ingredients in a blender.

5. Enjoy!

Calories: 271Fat: 3.7gCarbs: 54gProtein: 1.5g Fiber: 3.5g

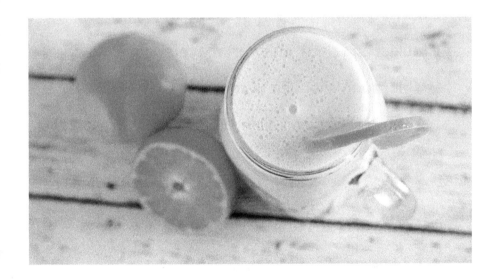

Creamy Relaxing Smoothie

Preparation Time: 13 minutes

Cooking Time: 15 Minutes

Serving: 3

Ingredients

1 cup soft-jelly coconut milk

1/4 seeded cucumber

1 Burro banana

1 tablespoon date sugar or agave syrup

1 tablespoon chopped walnuts

1/2 cup prepared Alkaline Diet's Nerve/Stress Relief Herbal Tea

1/4 avocado

Directions

1. Boil two cups of distilled water

2. Add a tablespoon of Alkaline Diet's Nerve Relief Herbal Tea.

3. Stir for 15 minutes, strain and let cool

4. Blend half a cup of the tea with what's left of the ingredients in a blender.

5. Add more sweetener if needed.

6. Enjoy your smoothie!

Calories: 271Fat: 4.7gCarbs: 44gProtein: 6.5g Fiber: 3.5g

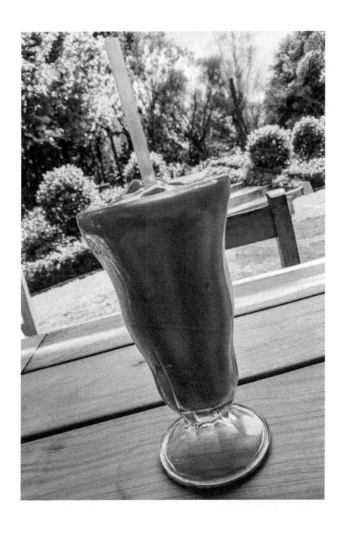

Nutmeg Green Beans

Preparation Time: 10 Minutes

Cooking Time: 30 Minutes

Servings: 4

Ingredients:

2 tablespoons olive oil

½ cup coconut cream

1-pound green beans, trimmed and halved

1 teaspoon nutmeg, ground

A pinch of salt and cayenne pepper

½ teaspoon onion powder

½ teaspoon garlic powder

2 tablespoons parsley, chopped

Directions:

Heat up a pan with the oil over medium heat, add the green beans, nutmeg and the other ingredients, toss, cook for 30 minutes, divide the mix between plates and serve.

Calories: 100 Cal

Fat: 13 g

Fiber: 2.3 g

Carbs: 5.1 g

Protein: 2 g

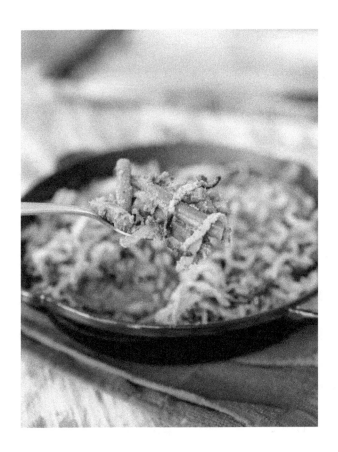

Cauliflower and Chives Mash

Preparation Time: 10 Minutes

Cooking Time: 20 Minutes

Servings: 4

Ingredients:

2 pounds cauliflower florets

2 cups water

1 teaspoon thyme, dried

1 teaspoon cumin, dried

1 cup coconut cream

2 garlic cloves, minced

A pinch of salt and black pepper

Directions:

Put the cauliflower florets in a pot, add the water and the other ingredients except the cream, bring to a simmer and cook over medium heat for 20 minutes.

Drain the cauliflower, add the cream, mash everything with a potato masher, whisk well, divide between plates and serve.

Calories: 200 Cal

Fat: 14.7 g

Fiber: 7.2 g

Carbs: 16.3 g

Protein: 6.1 g

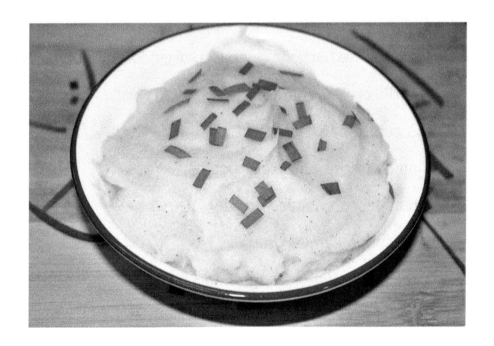

Baked Artichokes and Green Beans

Preparation Time: 10 Minutes

Cooking Time: 40 Minutes

Servings: 4

Ingredients:

1-pound green beans, trimmed and halved

3 scallions, chopped

2 tablespoons olive oil

1 cup canned artichoke hearts, drained and quartered

2 garlic cloves, minced

1/3 cup tomato passata

A pinch of salt and black pepper

2 teaspoons mustard powder

1 teaspoon cumin, ground

1 teaspoon coriander, ground

Directions:

Heat up a pan with the oil over medium heat, add the scallions and the garlic and sauté for 5 minutes.

Add the green beans and the other ingredients, toss, introduce in the oven and bake at 390 degrees F for 35 minutes.

Divide the mix between plates and serve as a side dish.

Calories: 132 Cal

Fat: 7.8 g Fiber: 6.9 g Carbs: 14.8 g Protein: 4.4 g

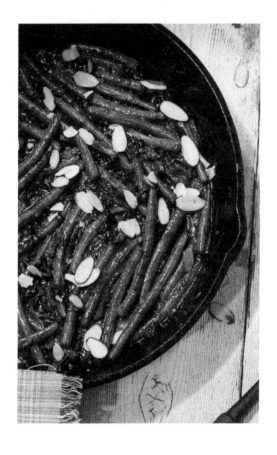

Cumin Cauliflower Rice and Broccoli

Preparation Time: 10 Minutes

Cooking Time: 25 Minutes

Servings: 4

Ingredients:

2 cups cauliflower rice

1 cup broccoli florets

2 tablespoons olive oil

4 scallions, chopped

1 teaspoon sweet paprika

1 teaspoon chili powder

1 cup vegetable stock

1 teaspoon red pepper flakes

A pinch of salt and black pepper

¼ teaspoon cumin, ground

Directions:

Heat up a pan with the oil over medium heat, add the scallions, paprika and chili powder and sauté for 5 minutes.

Add the cauliflower rice and the other ingredients, toss, bring to a simmer, cook over medium heat for 20 minutes, divide between plates and serve.

calories 81, fat 7.9, fiber 1.5, carbs 4.1, protein 1.1

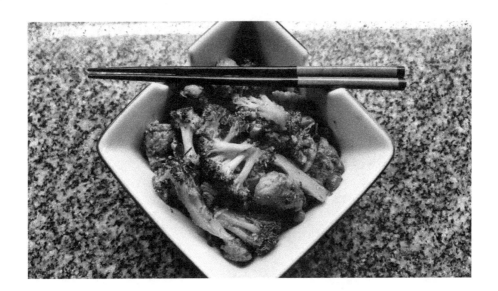

Flavored Tomato and Okra Mix

Preparation Time:

10 Minutes

Cooking Time:

30 Minutes

Servings: 6

Ingredients:

1 cup scallions, chopped

1-pound cherry tomatoes, halved

2 cups okra, sliced

2 tablespoons avocado oil

4 garlic cloves, chopped

2 teaspoons oregano, dried

A pinch of salt and black pepper

2 teaspoons cumin, ground

1 cup veggie stock

2 tablespoons tomato passata

Directions:

Heat up a pan with the oil over medium heat, add the scallions and the garlic and sauté for 5 minutes.

Add the tomatoes, the okra and the other ingredients, toss, cook over medium heat for 25 minutes, divide between plates and serve as a side dish.

Calories: 84 Cal

Fat: 2.1 g

Fiber: 5.4 g

Carbs: 14.8 g

Protein: 4 g

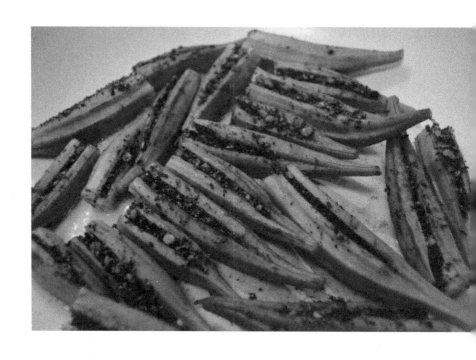

Roasted Artichokes and Sauce

Preparation Time: 10 Minutes

Cooking Time: 30 Minutes

Servings: 4

Ingredients:

2 big artichokes, trimmed and halved

2 tablespoons avocado oil

Juice of 1 lime

1 teaspoon turmeric powder

1 cup coconut cream

A pinch of salt and black pepper

½ teaspoon onion powder

¼ teaspoon sweet paprika

1 teaspoon cumin, ground

Directions:

In a roasting pan, combine the artichokes with the oil, the lime juice and the other ingredients, toss and bake at 390 degrees F for 30 minutes.

Divide the artichokes and sauce between plates and serve.

Calories: 190 Fat: 6 Fiber: 8 Carbs: 10 Protein: 9

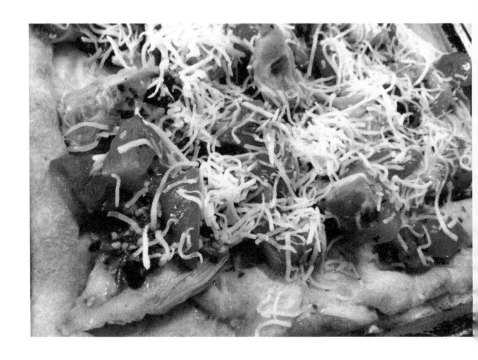

Zucchini Risotto

Preparation Time: 10 Minutes

Cooking Time: 30 Minutes

Servings: 4

Ingredients:

½ cup shallots, chopped

2 tablespoons olive oil

3 garlic cloves, minced

2 cups cauliflower rice

1 cup zucchinis, cubed

2 cups veggie stock

½ cup white mushrooms, chopped

½ teaspoon coriander, ground

A pinch of salt and black pepper

¼ teaspoon oregano, dried

2 tablespoons parsley, chopped

Directions:

Heat up a pan with the oil over medium heat, add the shallots, garlic, mushrooms, coriander and oregano, stir and sauté for 10 minutes.

Add the cauliflower rice and the other ingredients, toss, cook for 20 minutes more, divide between plates and serve.

Calories: 231 Cal Fat: 5 g Fiber: 3 g Carbs: 9 g Protein: 12 g

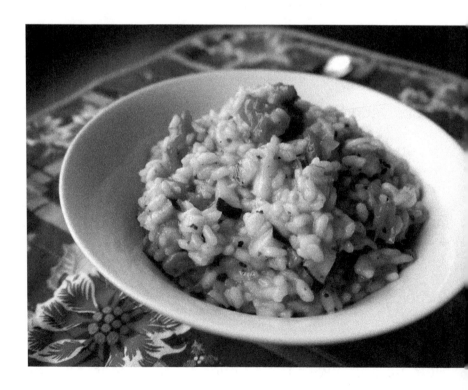

Cabbage and Rice

Preparation Time:

10 Minutes

Cooking Time:

30 Minutes

Servings: 4

Ingredients:

1 cup green cabbage, shredded

1 cup cauliflower rice

2 tablespoons olive oil

2 tablespoons tomato passata

2 spring onions, chopped

2 teaspoons balsamic vinegar

A pinch of salt and black pepper

2 teaspoons fennel seeds, crushed

1 teaspoon coriander, ground

Directions:

Heat up a pan with the oil over medium heat, add the spring onions, fennel and coriander, stir and cook for 5 minutes.

Add the cabbage, cauliflower rice and the other ingredients, toss, cook over medium heat for 25 minutes more, divide between plates and serve.

Calories: 200 Cal

Fat: 4 g

Fiber: 1 g

Carbs: 8 g

Protein: 5 g

Mini Turkey Meatloaves with Barbecue Sauce

Preparation Time: 7 Minutes

Cooking Time: 5 Minutes

Servings: 4

Ingredients

1 lb. ground turkey (not turkey breast)

1 small onion, cut into chunks, about 1/2 cup

1 celery rib, cut into a few large pieces

1/2 green bell pepper, about 1/4 cup

1 large egg, beaten with a splash of milk

3/4 cup breadcrumbs, plain

1/2 tablespoon McCormick's Montreal Brand steak seasoning

1/2 cup barbecue sauce

1/2 cup salsa

1 tablespoon Worcestershire sauce

 Olive oil

Directions

1. Preheat oven to 450 degrees and brush a 12-muffin tin with olive oil.

2. Put the ground turkey in a large bowl.

3. Put onion, celery and green pepper in the food processor. Pulse until finely chopped and add to the bowl of meat.

4. Add egg, breadcrumbs and steak seasoning to the bowl.

5. Mix together the BBQ sauce, salsa and Worcestershire in a separate small bowl. Pour half the sauce mixture into the bowl with the meat.

6. Mix the meatloaf together with your hands.

7. Using an ice cream scoop, fill the muffin tin and top each loaf with the remaining sauce.

8. Bake for 20 minutes.

Calories: 116 Cal

Fat: 21.3 g

Carbs: 5 g

Fiber: 2 g,

Protein: 4 g

Mixed Berry Crisp

Preparation Time: 10 Minutes

Cooking Time: 0

Servings: 4

Ingredients

1 1/2 cups mixed berries (I used raspberries, blueberries and blackberries)

1/2 tablespoon cornstarch

2 tablespoons butter, room temperature

1/4 cup old fashioned oats, plus 1 tablespoon old fashioned oats

1/4 cup brown sugar

3 tablespoons flour

1/4 teaspoon cinnamon

1/4 teaspoon nutmeg

1 tablespoon water

Directions

1. Preheat oven to 375 degrees.

2. Toss the berries with the cornstarch to evenly coat. Put the berry mixture in a large greased ramekin or a small greased baking dish (I used a 16 oz. ramekin).

3. In a small bowl, combine the butter, oats, brown sugar, flour, cinnamon and nutmeg. Mix lightly with a fork until the mixture is crumbly.

4. Top the berries with the crisp mixture. Sprinkle the top of the crisp with water.

5. Bake for 25 minutes or until the fruit is bubbling and the topping is slightly browned.

6. Serve with ice cream, frozen yogurt or whipped cream.

Calories: 226 Cal

Fat: 21.3 g

Carbs: 5 g

Fiber: 2 g,

Protein: 4 g

Orange Creamsicle Martini (Low Calorie!)

Preparation Time: 2 Minutes

Cooking Time: 0

Servings: 4

Ingredients

4 ounces diet orange soda, at room temperature

1 1/2 ounces orange-infused vodka (like Smirnoff Twist of Orange)

1 1/2 ounces torani sugar-free vanilla syrup

1 tablespoon Cool Whip Free

Directions

1. Place all ingredients in a martini shaker, but DO NOT shake (or the carbonated soda will explode!). Mix thoroughly with a spoon until mixture is mostly lump free. Add about 1 cup ice (crushed, if you have it), and stir until mixture is cold. Then place the strainer on top and pour into a large martini glass. Enjoy!

Calories: 116 Cal

Fat: 11.3 g

Carbs: 5 g

Fiber: 2 g,

Protein: 4 g

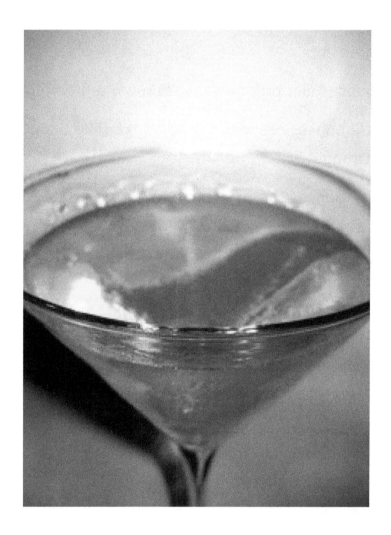

Adult Chocolate Milk with Spiced Rum

Preparation Time: 8 Minutes

Cooking Time: 15 Minutes

Servings: 4

Ingredients

2 ounces spiced rum

1 cup skim milk

1 tablespoon chocolate syrup

1/2 teaspoon vanilla

 Cola or diet cola

Directions

1. Add all ingredients except cola to a water bottle, drink mixer, or some other container with a lid.

2. Shake the hell out of it.

3. Pour into a glass and top off with cola. I use Diet Coke, and probably 1/2 cup of it, but for a sweeter drink, use more cola.

4. Drink.

5. Repeat several times.

Calories: 116 Cal

Fat: 21.3 g

Carbs: 5 g

Fiber: 2 g,

Protein: 4 g

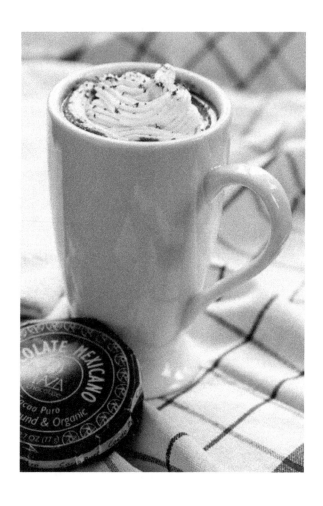

Strawberry Daiquiri
Preparation Time: 10 Minutes

Cooking Time: 24 Minutes

Servings: 4

Ingredients

1 (10 ounce) can froze strawberry daiquiri concentrate

1 (10 ounce) can froze strawberry daiquiri concentrate

1 1/2 cups frozen strawberries

1 cup ice cube

Directions

1. Combine all ingredients together in blender until all the ice is crushed.

2. Add more or less ice-cubes for the right texture.

Calories: 113 Cal

Fat: 21.3 g

Carbs: 5 g

Fiber: 2 g,

Protein: 4 g

Diabetic Virgin White Sangria

Preparation Time: 5 Minutes

Cooking Time: 4 Minutes

Servings: 1

Ingredients

4 cups ocean spray white cranberry juice with Splenda

2 cups fresh fruit, sliced

1 cup diet lemon-lime soda

1 lime, juice of

Directions

1. Combine all the ingredients except the soda in a large pitcher and chill for at least 1 hour.

2. When serving, add the soda. Serve with a pretty fruit garnish.

Calories: 126 Cal

Fat: 21.3 g

Carbs: 5 g

Fiber: 2 g,

Protein: 4 g

Wow Cola Chicken

Preparation Time: 15 Minutes

Cooking Time: 14 Minutes

Servings: 1

Ingredients

16 ounces boneless chicken breasts

1 (12 ounce) can diet cola

1 cup ketchup

Directions

1. Place chicken in crockpot and then top with ketchup and then pour cola over all.

2. Cook on low for 6-8 hours.

Calories: 306 Cal

Fat: 21.3 g

Carbs: 5 g

Fiber: 2 g,

Protein: 4 g

Yummy Berry Cooler

Preparation Time: 5 Minutes

Cooking Time: 4 Minutes

Servings: 1

Ingredients

2 2/3 cups cranberry-raspberry juice (I use the Splenda sweetened light version)

1 cup diet lemon-lime soda

Cool Whip

4 cherries

Directions

1. Combine first 3 ingredients.

2. Add ice if desired.

3. Top each glass with whipped cream and cherry.

Calories: 106 Cal

Fat: 21.3 g

Carbs: 3 g

Fiber: 1 g,

Protein: 4 g

Low Carb Sweet and Sour Chicken
Preparation Time: 15 Minutes

Cooking Time: 4 Minutes

Servings: 2

Ingredients

1 -11/2 lb. boneless chicken, cut up

1 cup white onion (you can leave the chunks big so you can pick them out)

12 ounces diet orange soda (Diet Rite Tangerine works great)

2 tablespoons soy sauce

2 tablespoons white vinegar

1 teaspoon ground ginger

1/2 teaspoon garlic powder

1/4teaspoon cayenne pepper

 Black pepper, to taste

Directions

1. Brown chicken and onions in a non-stick pan sprayed with cooking spray.

2. When chicken is brown, add the remaining ingredients.

3. Cover and simmer for about 20 minutes until the chicken is tender and thoroughly cooked.

4. Uncover and reduce liquid until it makes a syrupy sauce.

5. A little arrowroot powder may be added to thicken the sauce, if desired.

Calories: 106 Cal

Fat: 21.3 g

Carbs: 5 g

Fiber: 2 g,

Protein: 8 g

Warm Apple Delight

Preparation Time: 5 Minutes

Cooking Time: 4 Minutes

Servings: 1

Ingredients

2 red apples, cored & cut in half

1 (375 ml) canflavoured diet cola (cherry or strawberry suggested)

1 pinch Splenda sugar substitute or 1 pinch Equal sugar substitute

1 pinch cinnamon

Directions

1. Place the apple in a baking dish, skin side down and pour the cola over.

2. Sprinkle with sweetener & cinnamon.

3. Bake in a pre-heated oven at 180.C for 25-30 minutes.

Calories: 156 Cal

Fat: 21.3 g

Carbs: 5 g

Fiber: 2 g,

Protein: 4 g

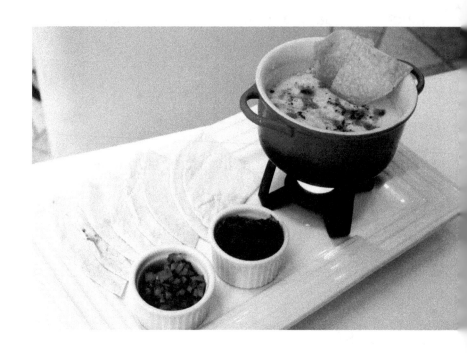

Orange Dream Cake

Preparation Time: 5 Minutes

Cooking Time: 4 Minutes

Servings: 1

Ingredients

18 1/4 ounces orange cake mix (1 box)

10 fluid ounces diet orange soda

2 egg whites

6 ounces sugar-free orange gelatin, divided (2 pkgs)

1 cup hot water

1 cup cold water

TOPPING

3 1/2 ounces fat-free sugar-free vanilla pudding mix

1 cup nonfat milk

1 teaspoon vanilla extract

8 ounces Cool Whip Free, thawed

Directions

1. Mix Cake mix, soda and egg whites together.

2. Pour batter into a 9 X 13 inch pan.

3. Bake as directed on box.

4. When done, use a meat fork to poke holes across the top of the entire cake.

5. Allow cake to cool.

6. In a medium bowl, mix together 1 box of the orange gelatin, 1 cup hot water and 1 cup cold water.

7. Pour gelatin mixture over top of cake.

8. Refrigerate for 2 to 3 hours.

9. Meanwhile, mix remaining box of jello, vanilla pudding mix, nonfat milk, and vanilla together. Beat well.

10. Fold whipped topping into this mixture, and spread on top of cake.

11. Chill in refrigerator until serving.

Calories: 106 Cal

Fat: 11.3 g

Carbs: 5 g

Fiber: 2 g,

Protein: 9 g

Capriosa De Fresca

Preparation Time:

5 Minutes

Cooking Time:

7 Minutes

Servings: 1

Ingredients

1 1/2 ounces strawberry vodka (Stoli, Smirnoff, etc)

7 ounces diet 7-Up (regular can be used if you prefer, also, if you want the drink to be less sweet, then substitute CLU)

3 fresh strawberries, sliced

2 slices limes (small wedges)

1 teaspoon sugar

Directions

1. Place the strawberries and lime wedges in the bottom of your cocktail glass. Muddle.

2. Add the strawberry vodka.

3. Add the 7-Up.

4. Gradually add the sugar to match your taste preference. (You can also add the sugar in the first step, this will make the fruit a little sweeter. I personally recommend this method if you like your drink to be a little on the sweet side.).

Calories: 216 Cal

Fat: 21.3 g

Carbs: 5 g

Fiber: 2 g,

Protein: 6 g

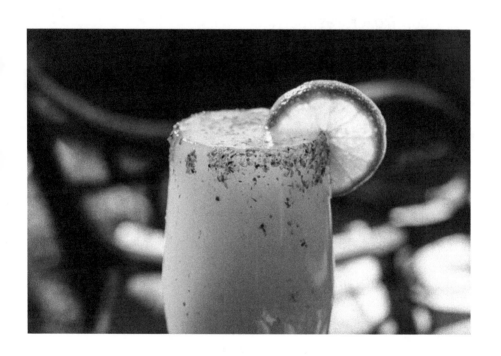

Delicious Low Cal Smoothie

Preparation Time: 5 Minutes

Cooking Time: 4 Minutes

Servings: 1

Ingredients

1 cup frozen raspberries

1 1/2 cups frozen strawberries

1 cup pineapple

355 ml diet Sprite

Directions

1. If your pineapple isn't already chopped up, chop it into pieces so it's easier to blend.

2. Add all fruits into a blender.

3. Add the can of sprite, add less than the whole can if you want a thicker smoothie.

4. Blend on high power until smooth.

5. Serve in your favorite glasses, either with spoons or straws.

Calories: 126 Cal

Fat: 21.3 g

Carbs: 5 g

Fiber: 2 g,

Protein: 4 g

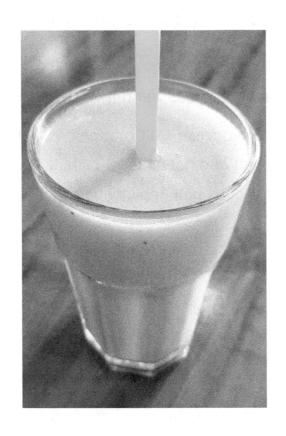

Diabetic Mock Sangria

Preparation Time: 5 Minutes

Cooking Time: 4 Minutes

Servings: 1

Ingredients

2 cups orange juice, chilled

1 cup unsweetened white grape juice, chilled

1 cup reduced-calorie cranberry juice cocktail

1 (1 liter) bottle diet lemon-lime soda, chilled ice cube

2 cups mixed fresh fruit oranges, cut into wedges, thinly sliced and halved or 2 cups lemons or 2 cups limes or 2 cups pineapple chunks

 Fresh mint sprig

Directions

1. In a large bowl or pitcher, stir together chilled orange juice, white grape juice, and cranberry juice.

2. Add the lemon-lime beverage; stir gently.

3. Fill each of 10 glasses about two-thirds full with ice.

4. Divide fruit among glasses.

5. Pour juice mixture into glasses and stir gently.

6.6. Ounce) servings.

Calories: 106 Cal

Fat: 21.3 g

Carbs: 5 g

Fiber: 2 g,

Protein: 4 g

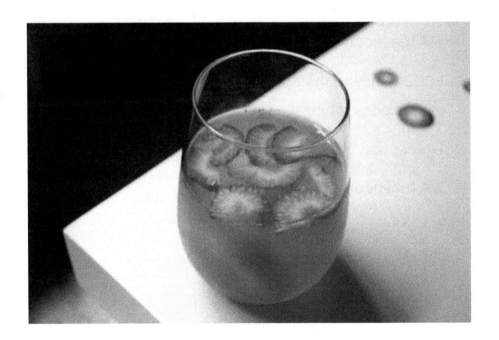

Slow Cooker 4th of July Chuck Roast Barbecue Sandwiches

Preparation Time: 15 Minutes

Cooking Time: 4 Minutes

Servings: 1

Ingredients

2 1/2 lbs. trimmed boneless chuck roast

2 chopped onions

1 (12 ounce) can diet cola

1/4 teaspoon Worcestershire sauce

1 1/2 tablespoons apple cider vinegar or 1 1/2 tablespoons white vinegar

1 teaspoon beef bouillon granules

3/4 teaspoon dry mustard

3/4 teaspoon chili powder

1/4-1/2teaspoon ground red pepper

3 cloves minced garlic

1 cup ketchup

1 tablespoon light butter

12 reduced-fat hamburger buns with sesame seeds

Directions

1. Place roast in a 3 1/2 or 4 quart electric slow cooker; add onion.

2. Combine cola and next 7 ingredients; cover and chill 1 cup sauce.

3. Pour remaining sauce over roast.

4. Cover with lid; cook on High for 1 hour.

5. Reduce heat to Low; cook 8 hours or until roast is very tender.

6. If time doesn't permit, you can omit cooking it on High for 1 hour.

7. Just add two hours to the Low cooking time.

8. Remove roast with chopped onion from cooker using a slotted spoon and shred meat with 2 forks.

9. Combine reserved sauce, ketchup and butter in a saucepan; cook over medium heat, stirring constantly, until thoroughly heated.

10. Pour sauce over shredded meat, stirring gently.

11. Spoon meat mixture on buns.

Calories: 122 Cal

Fat: 21.3 g

Carbs: 5 g

Fiber: 2 g,

Protein: 4 g

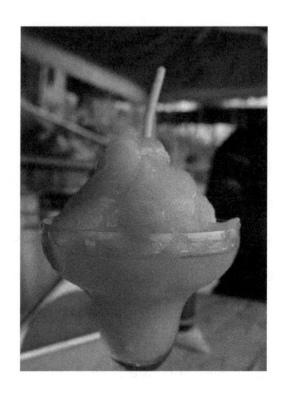

Berries Salad with Whipped Ricotta Cream

Preparation Time: 5 Minutes

Cooking Time: 4 Minutes

Servings: 1

Ingredients

2 cups strawberries, freshly sliced

1 cup blueberries

1/4 cup diet lemon-lime soda, divided

1 tablespoon fresh mint leaves, chopped

 1/2 cup skim milk ricotta cheese

2 1/2 teaspoons lemon zest

2 tablespoons nonfat sour cream

Directions

1. Toss strawberries, blueberries, 2 tablespoons of soda and mint together in a medium bowl; set aside for 10 minutes.

2. Meanwhile, combine ricotta, remaining 2 tablespoons of soda and lemon zest in another bowl.

3. Whip with a hand-held mixer until light and fluffy; stir in sour cream.

4. Place about 3/4 cup of berry mixture in each of 4 small bowls and top each serving with 1/3 cup of cream.

Calories: 119 Cal

Fat: 11.3 g

Carbs: 5 g

Fiber: 2 g,

Protein: 4 g

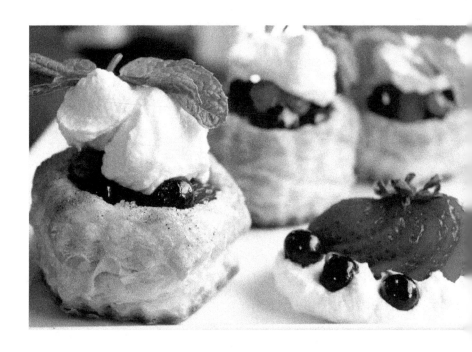

Seitan Tex-Mex Casserole

Preparation Time: 5 Minutes

Cooking Time: 35 Minutes

Servings: 4

Ingredients:

2 tbsp. vegan butter

1 ½ lb. seitan

3 tbsp. Tex-Mex seasoning

2 tbsp. chopped jalapeño peppers

½ cup crushed tomatoes

Salt and black pepper to taste

½ cup shredded vegan cheese

1 tbsp. chopped fresh green onion to garnish

1 cup sour cream for serving

Directions:

Preheat the oven and grease a baking dish with cooking spray. Set aside.

Melt the vegan butter in a medium skillet over medium heat and cook the seitan until brown, 10 minutes.

Stir in the Tex-Mex seasoning, jalapeño peppers, and tomatoes; simmer for 5 minutes and adjust the taste with salt and black pepper.

Transfer and level the mixture in the baking dish. Top with the vegan cheese and bake in the upper rack of the oven for 15 to 20 minutes or until the cheese melts and is golden brown.

Remove the dish and garnish with the green onion.

Serve the casserole with sour cream.

Calories: 464 Cal

Fat: 37.8 g

Carbs: 12 g

Fiber: 2 g

Protein: 24 g

Mushroom, Spinach and Turmeric Frittata

Preparation time: 10 minutes

Cooking time: 40 minutes

Servings: 6

Ingredients:

½ tsp. pepper

½ tsp. salt

1 tsp. turmeric

5-oz firm tofu

4 large eggs

6 large egg whites

¼ cup water

1 lb. fresh spinach

6 cloves freshly chopped garlic

1 large onion, chopped

1 lb. button mushrooms, sliced

Directions:

Grease a 10-inch nonstick and oven proof skillet and preheat oven to 350oF.

Place skillet on medium high fire and add mushrooms. Cook until golden brown.

Add onions, cook for 3 minutes or until onions are tender.

Add garlic, sauté for 30 seconds.

Add water and spinach, cook while covered until spinach is wilted, around 2 minutes.

Remove lid and continue cooking until water is fully evaporated.

In a blender, puree pepper, salt, turmeric, tofu, eggs and egg whites until smooth. Pour into skillet once liquid is fully evaporated.

Pop skillet into oven and bake until the center is set around 25-30 minutes.

Remove skillet from oven and let it stand for ten minutes before inverting and transferring to a serving plate.

Cut into 6 equal wedges, serve and enjoy.

Calories 358

Fat 6g

Carbs 65g

Protein 21g

Fiber 12g

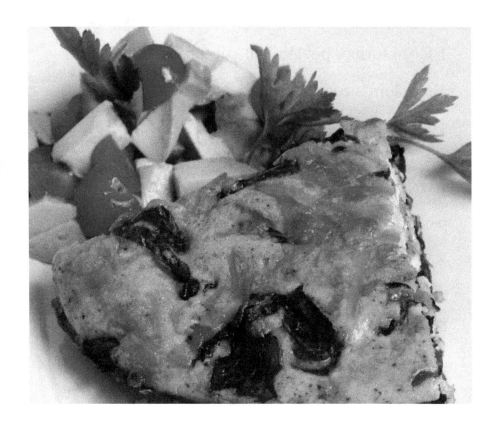

Roasted Root Vegetables

Preparation time: 10 minutes

Cooking time: 1 hour and 30 minutes

Servings: 6

Ingredients:

2 tbsp. olive oil

1 head garlic, cloves separated and peeled

1 large turnip, peeled and cut into ½-inch pieces

1 medium sized red onion, cut into ½-inch pieces

1 ½ lbs. beets, trimmed but not peeled, scrubbed and cut into ½-inch pieces

1 ½ lbs. Yukon gold potatoes, unpeeled, cut into ½-inch pieces

2 ½ lbs. butternut squash, peeled, seeded, cut into ½-inch pieces

Directions:

Grease 2 rimmed and large baking sheets. Preheat oven to 425oF.

In a large bowl, mix all ingredients thoroughly.

Into the two baking sheets, evenly divide the root vegetables, spread in one layer.

Season generously with pepper and salt.

Pop into the oven and roast for 1 hour and 15 minute or until golden brown and tender.

Remove from oven and let it cool for at least 15 minutes before serving.

Calories 278

Fat 5g

Carbs 57g

Protein 6g

Fiber 10g

Tropical Fruit Parfait

Preparation time: 10 minutes

Cooking time: 10 minutes

Servings: 1

Ingredients:

1 tbsp. toasted sliced almonds

¼ cup plain soy yogurt

½ cup of fruit combination cut into ½-inch cubes (pineapple, mango and kiwi)

Instructions:

Prepare fresh fruit by peeling and slicing into ½-inch cubes.

Place cubed fruit in a bowl and top with a dollop of soy yogurt.

Garnish with sliced almonds and if desired, refrigerate for an hour before serving.

Calories 119

Fat 2g

Carbs 25g

Protein 2g

Fiber 1g

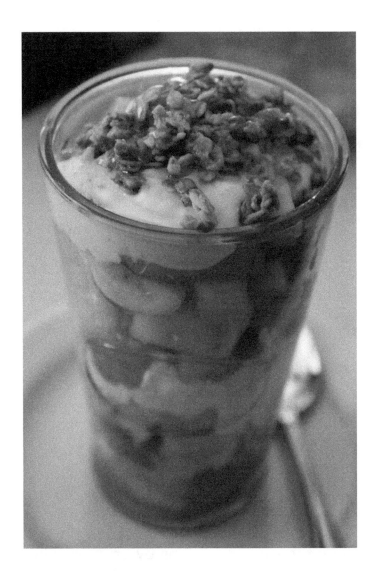

Cinnamon Chips with Avocado-Strawberry Salsa

Preparation time: 10 minutes

Cooking time: 10 minutes

Servings: 6

Ingredients:

3/8 tsp. salt

2 tsp. fresh lime juice

1 tsp. minced seeded jalapeno pepper

2 tbsp. minced fresh cilantro

1 cup finely chopped strawberries

1 ½ cups finely chopped, peeled and ripe avocado

½ tsp. ground cinnamon

2 tsp. sugar

6 6-inch brown rice tortillas

2 tsp. olive oil

Directions:

Preheat oven to 350oF.

Prepare the cinnamon chips by brushing olive oil all over the brown rice tortilla.

In a small bowl, mix together cinnamon and sugar.

Sprinkle cinnamon-sugar mixture evenly all over each of the brown rice tortilla.

Cut up each tortilla into 12 wedges, evenly and place on a baking sheet. If needed you can bake tortilla in two batches.

Pop the tortillas into the oven and bake until crisped, around 10 minutes. Remove from oven and keep warm.

Meanwhile, prepare salsa by mixing the remaining ingredients in a medium bowl. Stir to mix well.

To enjoy, dip crisped tortillas into bowl of salsa and eat or, you can spread the fruity salsa all over one tortilla chip and enjoy.

Calories 213

Fat 11g

Carbs 25g

Protein 5g

Fiber 7g

Stir Fried Brussels sprouts and Carrots

Preparation time: 10 minutes

Cooking time: 15 minutes

Servings: 6

Ingredients:

1 tbsp. cider vinegar

1/3 cup water

1 lb. Brussels sprouts, halved lengthwise

1 lb. carrots cut diagonally into ½-inch thick lengths

3 tbsp. olive oil, divided

2 tbsp. chopped shallot

½ tsp. pepper

¾ tsp. salt

Directions:

On medium high fire, place a nonstick medium fry pan and heat 2 tbsp. oil.

Ass shallots and cook until softened, around one to two minutes while occasionally stirring.

Add pepper salt, Brussels sprouts and carrots. Stir fry until vegetables starts to brown on the edges, around 3 to 4 minutes.

Add water, cook and cover.

After 5 to 8 minutes, or when veggies are already soft, add remaining butter.

If needed season with more pepper and salt to taste.

Turn off fire, transfer to a platter, serve and enjoy.

Calories 98

Fat 4g

Carbs 14g

Protein 3g

Fiber 5g

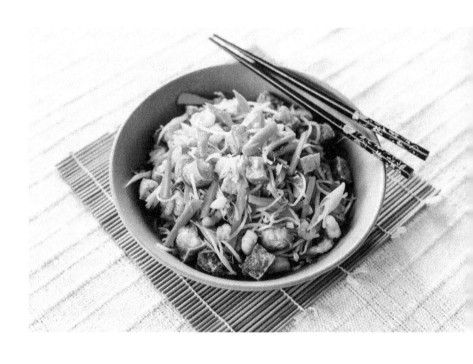

Curried Veggies and Poached Eggs

Preparation time: 10 minutes

Cooking time: 50 minutes

Servings: 4

Ingredients:

4 large eggs

½ tsp. white vinegar

1/8 tsp. crushed red pepper – optional

1 cup water

1 14-oz can chickpeas, drained

2 medium zucchinis, diced

½ lb. sliced button mushrooms

1 tbsp. yellow curry powder

2 cloves garlic, minced

1 large onion, chopped

2 tsp. extra virgin olive oil

Directions:

On medium high fire, place a large saucepan and heat oil.

Sauté onions until tender around four to five minutes.

Add garlic and continue sautéing for another half minute.

Add curry powder, stir and cook until fragrant around one to two minutes.

Add mushrooms, mix, cover and cook for 5 to 8 minutes or until mushrooms are tender and have released their liquid.

Add red pepper if using, water, chickpeas and zucchini. Mix well to combine and bring to a boil.

Once boiling, reduce fire to a simmer, cover and cook until zucchini is tender around 15 to 20 minutes of simmering.

Meanwhile, in a small pot filled with 3-inches deep of water, bring to a boil on high fire.

Once boiling, reduce fire to a simmer and add vinegar.

Slowly add one egg, slipping it gently into the water. Allow to simmer until egg is cooked, around 3 to 5 minutes.

Remove egg with a slotted spoon and transfer to a plate, one plate one egg.

Repeat the process with remaining eggs.

Once the veggies are done cooking, divide evenly into 4 servings and place one serving per plate of egg.

Serve and enjoy.

Calories 254

Fat 9g

Carbs 30g

Protein 16g

Fiber 9g

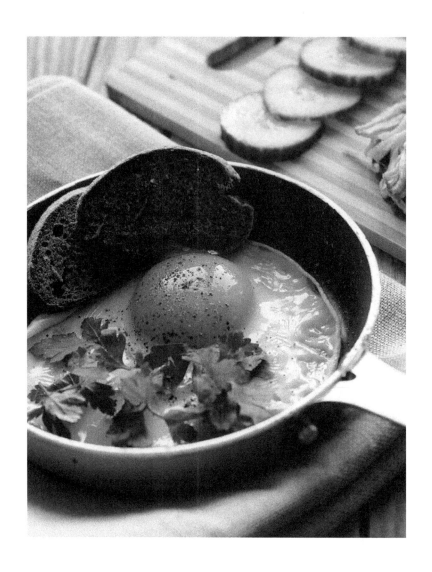

Braised Kale

Preparation Time: 10minutes

Cooking Time: 15 minutes

Servings 3

Ingredients:

2 to 3 tbsp. water

1 tbsp. coconut oil

½ sliced red pepper

2 stalk celery (sliced to ¼-inch thick)

5 cups of chopped kale

Directions:

Heat a pan over medium heat.

Add coconut oil and sauté the celery for at least five minutes.

Add the kale and red pepper.

Add a tablespoon of water.

Let the vegetables wilt for a few minutes. Add a tablespoon of water if the kale starts to stick to the pan.

Serve warm.

Calories 61

Fat 5g

Carbs 3g

Protein 1g

Fiber 1g,

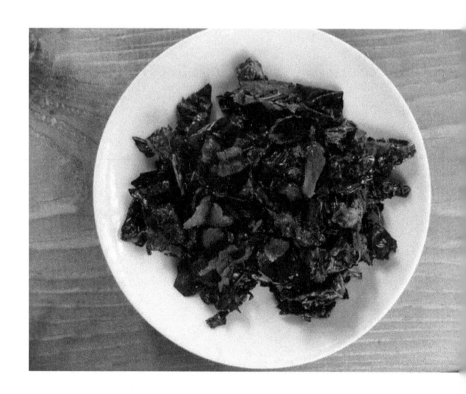

Braised Leeks, Cauliflower and Artichoke Hearts

Preparation Time: 10 minutes

Cooking Time: 10 minutes

Servings 4

Ingredients:

2 tbsp. coconut oil

2 garlic cloves, chopped

1 ½ cup artichoke hearts

1 ½ cups chopped leeks

1 ½ cups cauliflower flowerets

Directions:

Heat oil in a skillet over medium high heat.

Add the garlic and sauté for one minute. Add the vegetables and stir constantly until the vegetables are cooked.

Serve with roasted chicken, fish or pork.

Calories 111

Fat 7g

Carbs 12g

Protein 3g

Fiber 4g

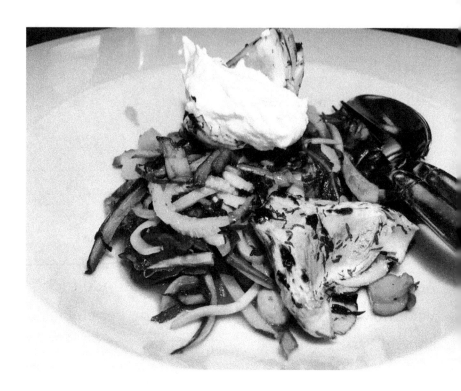

Celery Root Hash Browns

Preparation Time: 10 minutes

Cooking Time: 10 minutes

Servings 4

Ingredients:

4 tbsp. coconut oil

½ tsp. sea salt

2 to 3 medium celery roots

Directions:

Scrub the celery root clean and peel it using a vegetable peeler.

Grate the celery root in a food processor or a manual grater.

In a skillet, add oil and heat it over medium heat.

Place the grated celery root on the skillet and sprinkle with salt.

Let it cook for 10 minutes on each side or until the grated celery turns brown.

Serve warm.

Calories 160

Fat 14g

Fat 3g

Carbs 10g

Protein 1.5g

Fiber 3g

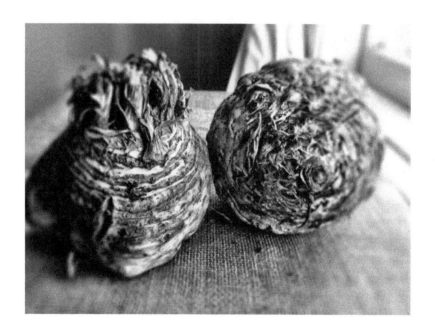

Zucchini Pasta with Avocado Sauce

Preparations Time: 10 minutes

Cooking Time: 10 minutes

Servings 1

Ingredients:

A squeeze of lemon juice

Salt and pepper to taste

1 tbsp. coconut milk

½ ripe avocado

1 medium zucchini cut into noodles

2 tbsp. olive oil

Directions:

Heat the oil in a skillet over medium heat and add the zucchini noodles. Sauté for three minutes or until the noodles have softened.

While the zucchini is cooking, mash the avocado together with the coconut milk, lemon juice and salt and pepper.

Add the sauce to the zucchini noodles and sauté. Serve warm.

Calories 471

Fat 43g

Carbs 23g

Protein 6g

Fiber 9g

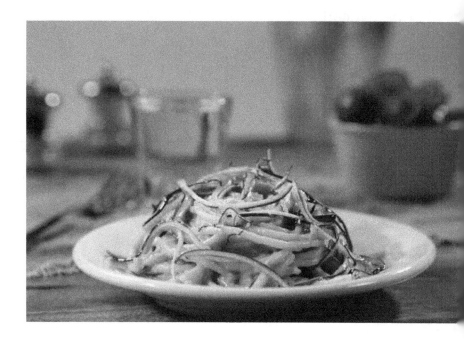

Zucchini Garlic Fries

Preparation Time: 10 minutes

Cooking Time: 20 minutes

Servings 6

Ingredients:

¼ teaspoon garlic powder

½ cup almond flour

2 large egg whites, beaten

3 medium zucchinis, sliced into fry sticks

Salt and pepper to taste

Directions:

Preheat oven to 400oF.

Mix all ingredients in a bowl until the zucchini fries are well coated.

Place fries on cookie sheet and spread evenly.

Put in oven and cook for 20 minutes.

Halfway through cooking time, stir fries.

Calories 11

Fat 0.1g,

Carbs 1g

Protein1.5 g

Fiber 0.5g

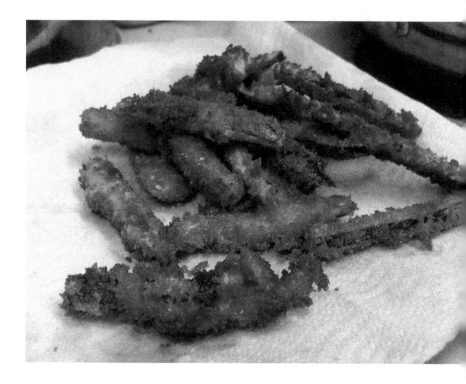

Avocado Coconut Pie

Preparation Time: 30 Minutes

Cooking Time: 50 Minutes

Servings: 4

Ingredients:

For the piecrust:

1 tbsp. flax seed powder + 3 tbsp. water

4 tbsp. coconut flour

4 tbsp. chia seeds

¾ cup almond flour

1 tbsp. psyllium husk powder

1 tsp. baking powder

1 pinch salt

3 tbsp. coconut oil

4 tbsp. water

For the filling:

2 ripe avocados

1 cup vegan mayonnaise

3 tbsp. flax seed powder + 9 tbsp. water

2 tbsp. fresh parsley, finely chopped

1 jalapeno, finely chopped

½ tsp. onion powder

¼ tsp. salt

½ cup cashew cream

1¼ cups shredded tofu cheese

Directions:

In 2 separate bowls, mix the different portions of flax seed powder with the respective quantity of water. Allow absorbing for 5 minutes.

Preheat the oven to 350 F.

In a food processor, add the coconut flour, chia seeds, almond flour, psyllium husk powder, baking powder, salt, coconut oil, water, and the smaller portion of the flax egg. Blend the ingredients until the resulting dough forms into a ball.

Line a spring form pan with about 12-inch diameter of parchment paper and spread the dough in the pan. Bake for 10 to 15 minutes or until a light golden brown color is achieved.

Meanwhile, cut the avocado into halves lengthwise, remove the pit, and chop the pulp. Put in a bowl and add the mayonnaise, remaining flax egg, parsley, jalapeno, onion powder, salt, cashew cream, and tofu cheese. Combine well.

Remove the piecrust when ready and fill with the creamy mixture. Level the filling with a spatula and continue baking for 35 minutes or until lightly golden brown.

When ready, take out. Cool before slicing and serving with a baby spinach salad.

Calories: 680 Cal

Fat: 71.8 g

Carbs: 10 g

Fiber: 7 g

Protein: 3 g

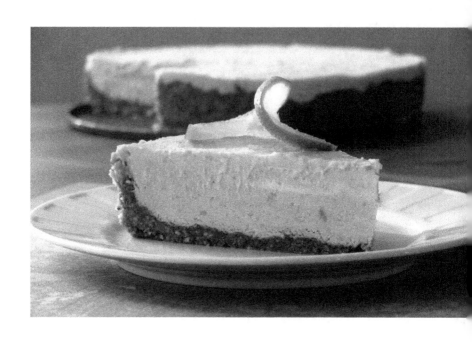

Baked Mushrooms with Creamy Brussels sprouts

Preparation Time: 8 Minutes

Cooking Time: 2 Hours 35 Minutes

Servings: 4

Ingredients:

For the mushrooms:

1 lb. whole white button mushrooms

Salt and black pepper to taste

2 tsp. dried thyme

1 bay leaf

5 black peppercorns

½ cups vegetable broth

2 garlic cloves, minced

1 ½ oz. fresh ginger, grated

1 tbsp. coconut oil

1 tbsp. smoked paprika

For the creamy Brussels sprouts:

½ lb. Brussels sprouts, halved

1 ½ cups cashew cream

Salt and ground black pepper to taste

Directions:

For the mushroom roast:

Preheat the oven to 200 F.

Pour all the mushroom ingredients into a baking dish, stir well, and cover with foil. Bake in the oven until softened, 1 to 2 hours.

Remove the dish, take off the foil, and use a slotted spoon to fetch the mushrooms onto serving plates. Set aside.

For the creamy Brussels sprouts:

Pour the broth in the baking dish into a medium pot and add the Brussels sprouts. Add about ½ cup of water if needed and cook for 7 to 10 minutes or until softened.

Stir in the cashew cream, adjust the taste with salt and black pepper, and simmer for 15 minutes.

Serve the creamy Brussels sprouts with the mushrooms.

Calories: 492 Cal

Fat: 37.9 g

Carbs: 13 g

Fiber: 2 g

Protein: 29 g

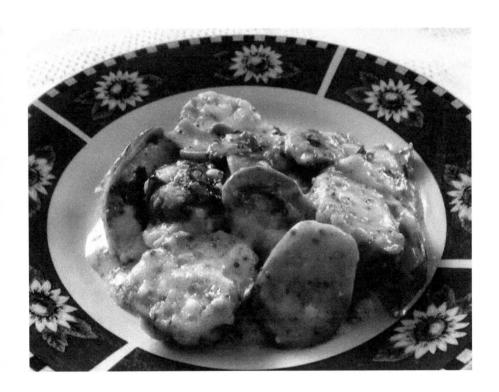

Pimiento Tofu balls

Preparation Time: 10 Minutes

Cooking Time: 15 Minutes

Servings: 4

Ingredients:

¼ cup chopped pimientos

1/3 cup mayonnaise

3 tbsp. cashew cream

1 tsp. paprika powder

1 pinch cayenne pepper

1 tbsp. Dijon mustard

4 oz. grated vegan cheese

1 ½ lbs. tofu, pressed and crumbled

Salt and black pepper to taste

2 tbsp. olive oil, for frying

Directions:

In a large bowl, add all the ingredients except for the olive oil and with gloves on your hands, mix the ingredients until well combined. Form bite size balls from the mixture.

Heat the olive oil in a medium non-stick skillet and fry the tofu balls in batches on both sides until brown and cooked through, 4 to 5 minutes on each side.

Transfer the tofu balls to a serving plate and serve warm.

Calories: 254 Cal

Fat: 36.8 g

Carbs: 12 g

Fiber: 1 g

Protein: 26 g

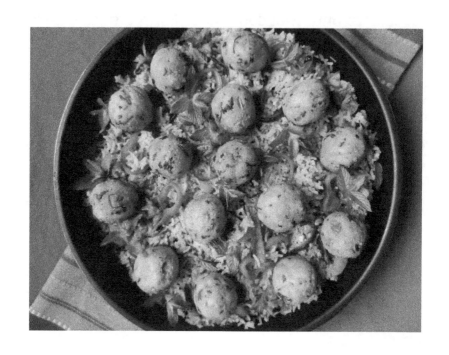

Tempeh with Garlic Asparagus

Preparation Time: 10 Minutes

Cooking Time: 18 Minutes

Servings: 4

Ingredients:

For the tempeh:

3 tbsp. vegan butter

4 tempeh slices

Salt and black pepper to taste

For the garlic buttered asparagus:

2 tbsp. olive oil

2 garlic cloves, minced

1 lb. asparagus, trimmed and halved

Salt and black pepper to taste

1 tbsp. dried parsley

1 small lemon, juiced

Directions:

For the tempeh:

Melt the vegan butter in a medium skillet over medium heat, season the tempeh with salt, black pepper and fry in the butter on both sides until brown and cooked through, 10 minutes. Transfer to a plate and set aside in a warmer for serving.

For the garlic asparagus:

Heat the olive oil in a medium skillet over medium heat, and sauté the garlic until fragrant, 30 seconds.

Stir in the asparagus, season with salt and black pepper, and cook until slightly softened with a bit of crunch, 5 minutes.

Mix in the parsley, lemon juice, toss to coat well, and plate the asparagus.

Serve the asparagus warm with the tempeh.

Calories: 181

Fat: 17.5 g

Carbs: 6 g

Fiber: 3 g

Protein: 3 g

Mushroom Curry Pie

Preparation Time: 15 Minutes

Cooking Time: 55 Minutes

Servings 4

Ingredients:

For the piecrust:

1 tbsp. flax seed powder + 3 tbsp. water

¾ cup coconut flour

4 tbsp. chia seeds

4 tbsp. almond flour

1 tbsp. psyllium husk powder

1 tsp. baking powder

1 pinch salt

3 tbsp. olive oil

4 tbsp. water

For the filling:

1 cup chopped criminal mushrooms

1 cup vegan mayonnaise

3 tbsp. + 9 tbsp. water

½ red bell pepper, finely chopped

1 tsp. turmeric powder

½ tsp. paprika powder

½ tsp. garlic powder

¼ tsp. black pepper

½ cup cashew cream

1¼ cups shredded tofu cheese

Directions:

In two separate bowls, mix the different portions of flax seed powder with the respective quantity of water and set aside to absorb for 5 minutes.

Preheat the oven to 350 F.

Make the crust:

When the flax egg is ready, pour the smaller quantity into a food processor, and add the coconut flour, chia seeds, almond flour, psyllium husk powder, baking powder, salt, olive oil, and water. Blend the ingredients until a ball forms out of the dough.

Line a spring form pan with an 8-inch diameter parchment paper and grease the pan with cooking spray.

Spread the dough in the bottom of the pan and bake in the oven for 15 minutes.

Make the filling:

In a bowl, add the remaining flax egg, mushrooms, mayonnaise, water, bell pepper, turmeric, paprika, garlic powder, black pepper, cashew cream, and tofu cheese. Combine the mixture evenly and fill the piecrust. Bake further for 40 minutes or until the pie is golden brown.

Remove, slice, and serve the pie with a chilled strawberry drink.

Calories: 548 Cal

Fat: 55.9 g

Carbs: 6 g

Fiber: 2 g

Protein: 8 g

Spicy Cheese with Tofu Balls

Preparation Time: 20 Minutes

Cooking Time: 20 Minutes

Servings: 4

Ingredients:

For the spicy cheese:

1/3 cup vegan mayonnaise

¼ cup pickled jalapenos

1 tsp. paprika powder

1 tbsp. mustard powder

1 pinch cayenne pepper

4 oz. grated tofu cheese

For the tofu balls:

1 tbsp. flax seed powder + 3 tbsp. water

2 ½ cup crumbled tofu

Salt and black pepper

2 tbsp. plant butter, for frying

Directions:

Make the spicy cheese. In a bowl, mix the mayonnaise, jalapenos, paprika, mustard powder, cayenne powder, and cheddar cheese. Set aside.

In another medium bowl, combine the flax seed powder with water and allow absorbing for 5 minutes.

Add the flax egg to the cheese mixture, the crumbled tofu, salt, and black pepper, and combine well. Use your hands to form large meatballs out of the mix.

Then, melt the vegan butter in a large skillet over medium heat and fry the tofu balls until cooked and browned on the outside.

Serve the tofu balls with roasted cauliflower mash and mayonnaise.

Calories: 259 Cal

Fat: 55.9 g

Carbs: 5 g

Fiber: 1 g

Protein: 16 g

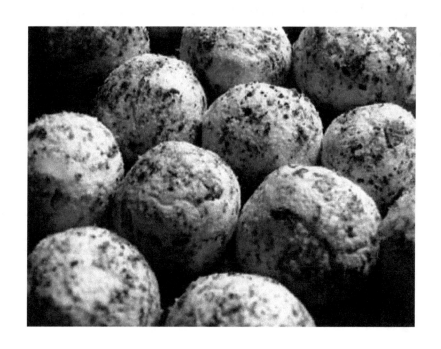

Tempeh Coconut Curry Bake

Preparation Time: 7minutes

Cooking Time: 23minutes

Servings: 4

Ingredients:

1 oz. plant butter, for greasing

2 ½ cups chopped tempeh

Salt and black pepper

4 tbsp. plant butter

2 tbsp. red curry paste

1 ½ cup coconut cream

½ cup fresh parsley, chopped

15 oz. cauliflower, cut into florets

Directions:

Preheat the oven to 400 F and grease a baking dish with 1 ounce of vegan butter.

Arrange the tempeh in the baking dish, sprinkle with salt and black pepper, and top each tempeh with a slice of the remaining butter.

In a bowl, mix the red curry paste with the coconut cream and parsley. Pour the mixture over the tempeh.

Bake in the oven for 20 minutes or until the tempeh is cooked.

While baking, season the cauliflower with salt, place in a microwave-safe bowl, and sprinkle with some water. Steam in the microwave for 3 minutes or until the cauliflower is soft and tender within.

Remove the curry bake and serve with the caulis.

Calories: 417 Cal

Fat: 38.8 g

Carbs: 11 g

Fiber: 2 g

Protein: 11 g

Printed in the USA
CPSIA information can be obtained
at www.ICGtesting.com
LVHW011029150224
771954LV00003B/8